MW00533901

The Effective Nurse Preceptor Training Handbook:

Your guide to success

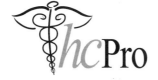

The Effective Nurse Preceptor Handbook: Your guide to success is published by HCPro, Inc.

Copyright 2003 HCPro, Inc.

HCPro provides information resources for the health care industry.

HCPro is not affiliated in any way with the Joint Commission on Accreditation of Healthcare Organizations, which owns the JCAHO trademark.

Brian R. Rogers, RN, BSc, CCRN, DHA, EMT-HP, Author
John Gettings, Associate Editor
Leah Tracosas, Copy Editor
Jean St. Pierre, Creative Director
Mike Mirabello, Senior Graphic Artist
Matthew Sharpe, Graphic Artist
Kathryn Levesque, Group Publisher
Suzanne Perney, Publisher

Advice given is general. Readers should consult professional counsel for specific legal, ethical, or clinical questions.

Arrangements can be made for quantity discounts.

For more information, contact:

HCPro
P.O. Box 1168
Marblehead, MA 01945
Telephone: 800/650-6787 or 781/639-1872
Fax: 781/639-2982
E-mail: *customerservice@hcpro.com*

Visit HCPro at its World Wide Web sites:
www.hcmarketplace.com, www.hcpro.com, and *www.himinfo.com.*

09/2003
19631

Contents

About the expert

Brian R. Rogers, RN, BSc, CCRN, DHA, EMT-HP

Brian R. Rogers, RN, BSc, CCRN, DHA, EMT-HP, has been a nurse and educator for over 25 years. He is a leading authority on cardiology-related program design and education.

Since graduating from the University of Toronto and the University of Saskatchewan in Canada, Rogers has had nursing experience in emergency room, intensive care unit, cardiac care unit, and post-anesthesia care unit, as well as experience as a transport paramedic. He has served as a director of nursing and a director of education in both large and small hospitals in both the United States and Canada. In addition, he has taught nursing at the community college level for several years.

Rogers has created more than 20 continuing education programs for nurses, including courses on critical-thinking skills for nurses, empowerment of the charge nurse, and preceptorship. He has published articles in many publications, including the Canadian Association of Quality Assurance Professionals' *Quality Assurance Quarterly, The Canadian Nurse,* and *The Official Journal of the Canadian Intravenous Nurses Association.* Rogers was founding president of the Canadian Association of Quality Assurance Professionals in 1980.

The Effective Nurse Preceptor Training Handbook:

Your guide to success

Wearing the preceptor hat

An effective preceptor, it has been reported, is one of the major factors that will affect the retention of a new nurse. The right preceptor can help the new nurse or graduate to overcome the hurdles of new technology, inadequate staffing, complicated medical interventions, and complex diagnoses.

For a nursing student or a new nurse practitioner, the ability to interact with a preceptor is vital to the effective learning of professional nursing practice. Functioning under the guidance of an effective preceptor will give the student nurse or novice an opportunity to experience direct nursing practice with expert guidance and support.

This handbook will provide you with the background necessary for helping the student or novice examine and apply nursing theory in a real practice setting, increasing personal and professional growth, and easing the transition into professional practice.

What is a preceptor?

A preceptor is a

- teacher
- coach
- cheerleader
- socializer
- recordkeeper
- evaluator
- advocate
- role model

Essential responsibilities of the preceptor

If you are to be all of these things, you must be willing to take on the following 12 essential responsibilities:

1. Orient your preceptee to the nursing unit. This will require a detailed orientation process that incorporates the physical layout of the unit as well as the unit's policies and procedures. Keep in mind the following points to help ensure that your preceptee gets the very best orientation:

   - Put yourself in his or her shoes
   - Acknowledge his or her presence
   - Talk about what's happening today
   - Introduce your orientee to your customers

- Give clear instructions
- Never abandon your orientee
- Help your orientee develop critical thinking skills
- Clue your orientee in to the chain of command
- Be positive
- Practice what you preach

2. Facilitate the learning experience. Facilitating learning is not simply a skill, such as administering an injection, which is the learning of a series of steps. Facilitating learning is making learning easier for your preceptee by providing support that will enable him or her to come into the workplace daily with a positive attitude, have correct behaviors reinforced and poor behaviors modified, and practice skills until they are mastered.

   This art of facilitation requires that you reflect on your own attitudes, behaviors, and skills. Ask yourself, "Am I able to model expert practice in the clinical setting daily?" Your preceptee has read about practice, discussed it in class, and observed it. Now he or she needs your support to apply his or her knowledge daily in professional practice and must be encouraged for doing so.

3. Establish the schedule for your preceptee and assistant preceptor. The focus of the preceptorship program is on individualized teaching and learning, role modeling, and the use of knowledge and practice of skills.

Your schedule should be prepared for the duration of the intended preceptorship period. Any potential scheduling conflicts with your preceptee should be discussed and applied to the process with the intent that you will spend as much time with your preceptee as possible.

If there are any scheduled shifts on which you and your preceptee cannot be matched, schedule your preceptee with an assistant preceptor.

4. Guide your preceptee during clinical practice. Be prepared to provide one-on-one guidance through the initial clinical practice. This responsibility should involve the following:

   - Demonstration of nursing skills and techniques
   - Supervised clinical practice of those skills and techniques at the bedside
   - Competency validation once sufficient practice has become a mastered skill

   Always keep in mind that patient safety and comfort is paramount. Thus, interventions during practice should be limited to situations in which a danger to the patient exists.

   Avoid stepping in to speed up the process or to do it "your way." Preceptors should remember the adage, "Thou shalt not make a clone of thyself."

5. Supervise competency validation during clinical practice.

An important factor of this responsibility is your ability to give directions. Read the following four tips for guidance on giving directions to orientees:

1. Don't assume they're familiar with the situation. Find out what they know before discussing what they need to know.

2. Encourage them to clarify your instructions by asking questions. Reassure them that no question is off-limits (e.g., "There's no such thing as a stupid question").

3. Ask questions to confirm their comprehension. Most people won't admit they don't understand instructions.

4. Always include a "why" with directions, no matter how brief. Your new staff will carry out the task correctly if they understand why they're doing it in the first place.

Competency validation should follow the organization's policies for this process. In general, competency can be defined as the ability to perform a process or procedure according to generally accepted standards for practice. It is important that a list of competencies for each preceptee be established. Each day, choose assignments that will give your preceptee the necessary clinical practice and supervision to eventually be "checked-off" on each competency.

6. Teach new skills and reinforce previous learning. Nursing is a practice-based profession, and the quality of clinical education is paramount to establishing a successful nursing career. Teach or reinforce the new skills that your preceptee has not had a chance to practice (or even a chance to learn in the first place) and the theory behind those skills.

   First, establish what your preceptee already knows or can do, demonstrate the new skills, and have he or she perform a return demonstration. Then evaluate the outcome from the new skill or process as it is applied at the bedside.

7. Gradually increase your preceptee's responsibility for patient care. Usually, new nurses or students will have had the opportunity to provide care for only one or two patients. Most medical-surgical units will require the new employee to care for between six and eight patients. It is a tough transition for a preceptee to make without guidance on how to set priorities, establish daily goals, manage time well, and communicate effectively to other team members. By gradually introducing new patients, you will help your new nurse focus on these areas of learning.

8. Provide timely feedback to your preceptee regarding all aspects of clinical practice. Feedback needs to be given as

events occur during the orientation process. This feedback should serve two purposes: It should reinforce positive behavior, as well as promptly extinguish inappropriate behaviors. A quiet, private setting is needed to ensure that you do not hurt your preceptee's ego. (Note: There is more guidance on giving feedback beginning on p. 30.)

9. Serve as a role model for your preceptee during clinical experiences. This requirement will be the hardest for many preceptors. Consistently present many of the positive attributes that helped you become a candidate for preceptorship. There are also subtle role-modeling techniques to remember, such as the following:

   - Keep professional uniforms
   - Maintain excellent attendance
   - Arrive to work early
   - Be prepared for report
   - Follow institutional policy/procedure at all times
   - Express positive comments during staff meetings
   - Be a member in a professional organization such as the Emergency Nurses Association or the American Association of Critical Care Nurses

10. Work closely with nursing faculty/the hospital educator to identify education gaps and learning opportunities. Often it will be beyond your scope to accomplish more complex training needs. For example, if you participate in a preceptorship program on a progressive care unit that

requires knowledge and skill in electrocardiogram (ECG) rhythm interpretation, then you might wish to discuss learning opportunities with the hospital educator, who may have classes planned. It would be then your job to validate the learning with patient care activities involving ECG rhythm-strip interpretation and the clinical impact on the patient.

11. Plan specific learning experiences that correlate with unit competencies and clinical objectives. You may have to plan mock experiences that will mimic the unit requirements for patient care. Examples include cardiac arrest, disaster response, and use of equipment that is infrequently applied during patient care. The goal is to ensure that your preceptee has as many opportunities for supervised practice of the wide variety of skills needed for the particular nursing unit. Any skill that has a low frequency of use, but a high probability of potential harm to the patient if done incorrectly, must have the competency validated by you, if possible.

12. Complete all necessary paperwork related to the preceptor program. The timely completion of forms, checklists, and evaluations ensures that communication regarding the progress of the preceptee toward independent practice is happening on schedule.

Expectations of the preceptor

You are fulfilling your role and responsibilities as preceptor if you are doing the following:

1. Working collaboratively with each of the following:

   - Manager
   - Educator
   - Preceptee
   - Faculty member (if applicable)

2. Organizing learning experiences
3. Acting as an advocate by doing the following:

   - Initiating introductions
   - Identifying resource materials
   - Answering questions
   - Solving problems

Understanding adult learning

"Thou shalt not make a clone of thyself." This saying is a quick reminder that the way you may have learned how to do something isn't the only way that process can be done. If a student learns another way of doing a task, yet the end result is the same, you should be satisfied. Remember that there's more than one way to get things done.

Use adult learning principles to examine the way you teach and others learn to ensure that you can identify and account for differences.

Identifying learning styles

To understand how to teach others, you must have an understanding of the variety of ways that people learn. Complete the "Learning style inventory test" on pp. 11–12 and then score the test using the "Scoring procedures" guide on p. 13.

Are you a visual, auditory, or tactile learner? Do you see the implications that each learning style may have for the orientee's training process?

Learning style inventory test

To gain a better understanding of yourself as a learner, you need to evaluate the way you prefer to learn or process information. By doing so, you will be able to develop strategies that will enhance both your learning and teaching potential.

This 24-item survey is not timed. Answer each question as honestly as you can.

Place a ✓ on the appropriate line after each statement.

	Often	Sometimes	Seldom
1. Can remember more about a subject through the lecture method, with information, explanations, and discussion.			
2. Prefer information to be written on the chalkboard, with the use of visual aids and assigned readings.			
3. Like to write things down or to take notes for visual review.			
4. Prefer to use posters, models, actual practice, and some activities in class.			
5. Require explanations of diagrams, graphs, or visual directions.			
6. Enjoy working with my hands or making things.			
7. Am skillful with, and enjoy developing and making, graphs and charts.			
8. Can tell whether sounds match when presented with pairs of sounds.			
9. Remember best by writing things.			
10. Can understand and follow directions on maps.			
11. Do better at academic subjects by listening to lectures and tapes.			
12. Play with coins or keys in pockets.			

Learning style inventory test (cont.)

	Often	Sometimes	Seldom
13. Learn to spell better by repeating the words out loud than by writing the word on paper.			
14. Can better understand a news article by reading about it in the paper than by listening to the radio.			
15. Chew gum, smoke, or snack during studies.			
16. Feel the best way to remember is to picture it in my head.			
17. Learn spelling by "finger spelling" words.			
18. Would rather listen to a good lecture or speech than read about the same material in a textbook.			
19. Am good at working and solving jigsaw puzzles and mazes.			
20. Grip objects in hands during learning period.			
21. Prefer listening to the news on the radio rather than reading about it in the newspaper.			
22. Obtain information on an interesting subject by reading relevant materials.			
23. Feel very comfortable touching others, hugging, handshaking, and so on.			
24. Follow oral directions better than written ones.			

Scoring procedures

Scoring Procedures

Please insert the following point values on the line next to the corresponding item. Add the points in each column to obtain the total preference scores under each heading.

Often = 5 points   Sometimes = 3 points   Seldom = 1 point

Visual		Auditory		Tactile	
No.	Pts.	No.	Pts.	No.	Pts.
2.		1.		4.	
3.		5.		6.	
7.		8.		9.	
10.		11.		12.	
14.		13.		15.	
16.		18.		17.	
19.		21.		20.	
22.		24.		23.	
Total VPS		Total APS		Total TPS	

VPS = Visual Preference Score
APS = Auditory Preference Score
TPS = Tactile Preference Score

If your VSP total was highest, you are a VISUAL learner.
Advice: Be sure that you look at all study materials. Use charts, maps, videos, notes, and flash cards. Practice visualizing or picturing words/concepts in your head. Write out everything for frequent and quick visual review.

If your APS total was highest, you are an AUDITORY learner.
Advice: You may wish to use tape recordings. Tape lectures to help you fill in the gaps in your notes. But do listen and take notes, and review those notes frequently. Sit somewhere in the lecture hall or classroom where you can hear well. After you have read something, summarize it and recite it aloud.

If your TPS total was highest, you are a TACTILE learner.
Advice: Trace words as you are saying them. For facts that must be learned, you should write them out several times. Keep a supply of scratch paper for this purpose. Taking and keeping lecture notes will be very important. Make study sheets.

For example, a basic understanding of policies used within the organization is required of nursing students and new employees. A **visual** learner may be able to read the policies and understand them. An **auditory** learner may need to have the policies read out loud and discussed. A **tactile** learner may have to actually implement the policies—in other words, do something—to fully grasp the policies.

Domains of learning

There are three learning domains: the cognitive domain, the psychomotor domain, and the affective domain. Each time you begin a teaching session, the domain in which you are teaching must be considered.

Cognitive domain

The cognitive domain is knowledge-based. It has three practical instructional levels: fact, understanding, and application.

1. The fact level is a single concept. To describe it, one would use verbs such as "define," "identify," or "list."
2. The understanding level puts two or more concepts together. Thus, to describe understanding, one would use verbs such as "describe," "compare," and "contrast."
3. The application level puts two or more concepts together to form something new. Usually descriptive verbs, including "explain," "apply," and "analyze," signal a move to the application level.

To teach subjects within the cognitive domain, use lectures, presentations, and written materials. To test retention within the cognitive domain, use both objective and subjective test items. For example, an objective test item might be asking your preceptee to calculate a drug dose, while a subjective test item would be asking your preceptee to choose an accurate pain description on a patient pain scale.

Psychomotor domain

The psychomotor domain is skill-based. Within this domain, the orientee or nursing student will produce a "product" of his or her skills at the bedside. The following are three practical instructional levels:

1. The first level, imitation, can be associated with demonstration delivery. That is, imitation will simply be a return demonstration under the watchful eye of the preceptor.
2. The practice level will be a proficiency-building experience that may be conducted by the preceptee without the direct oversight of the preceptor.
3. The habit level is reached when the orientee can perform the skill in twice the time that it takes the preceptor (an expert) to perform it.

To teach within the psychomotor domain, the preceptor will need to use performance skill testing.

Affective domain

The affective domain is based upon behavioral aspects, and it may be considered beliefs or values.

The three levels of the affective domain are awareness, distinction, and integration. The verbs that describe this domain are words such as "display," "exhibit," and "accept." This domain requires knowledge and the ability to distinguish when that knowledge should be used to accomplish a certain objective.

The preceptor must hold discussions to teach within this domain.

The ten principles of learning

Take a look at the following list of the 10 principles of learning. Each of the following principles precedes an appropriate application of that principle to the preceptorship program:

1. We learn by doing.
Allow the novice to do the task, no matter how slowly.

2. We learn by focusing on one task.
Focus on developing a single task each day.

3. We must be ready to learn new material/tasks.
Assess your preceptee to determine a readiness to learn new material.

4. We must be motivated to learn.
Encourage your orientee each time a task is accomplished.

5. We must have immediate reinforcement of learning.

Discuss the learning experience and its value to your preceptee.

6. **The learning situation must have meaningful content.**
   The planned learning experiences must relate directly to the care processes on the unit.

7. **Practice exercises must be as real as possible.**
   You may need to use a mannequin to simulate learning.

8. **Responses to the learning situation will vary.**
   You may have a different perception of a learning experience than your preceptee, but the one that counts is that of the preceptee.

9. **The learning atmosphere will have an impact.**
   When you allow your preceptee to make mistakes without humiliation, trust will ensue.

10. **Backgrounds and physical abilities will vary.**
    You will have different dexterity skills than the preceptee.

Creating a climate for learning

Establish a learning climate on the nursing unit that will help you implement the adult learning principles.

Physical challenges

The unit environment has to be consciously shaped to maximize personal interaction and learning. There must be suitable places for quiet reading, one-on-one discussions, small class settings, and practice space for demonstrations using mannequins or models. For longer sessions, it would be appropriate for refreshments to be made available.

Emotional challenges

The creation of a non-threatening emotional climate is a little more challenging and will take a little more time for you to achieve. The emotional climate will serve as a comfort zone, where everyone understands that every person's views are valued and respected as equal. How each member of the unit staff speaks to others in the group is important, as is full unit participation. One way to test the emotional climate is to encourage your preceptee to bring up subjects or ideas for discussion during staff meetings.

Helping new nurses overcome 'reality shock'

One of the major problems for health care institutions is the loss of new staff during the first six months of their employment. This group is made up of new graduates as well as seasoned professionals who are disillusioned with the modern health care work environment. This disillusionment is commonly known as "reality shock." Reality shock occurs when preceptees realize that the actual job is different than the one they thought they were preparing for.

This disparity often arises when ethical, moral, professional, or cultural beliefs of your preceptee conflict with the beliefs held by the nursing and allied health staff of the health care institution. A conflict may arise regarding work issues that causes so much anxiety your preceptee cannot perform his or her duties, and resigns to avoid the conflict.

Therefore, it is essential that you are familiar with the ethical, moral, professional, and cultural beliefs held by the institution and those held by your preceptee. This will help you guide your preceptee through the four phases of transition from preceptee to active staff member, while softening the blow of reality shock.

The four phases of workplace acclimation

There are four phases that many preceptees experience during the first six months of employment. In chronological order, they are as follows:

1. The honeymoon phase
2. The shock phase
3. The recovery phase
4. The resolution phase

The honeymoon phase

During the honeymoon phase your preceptee is likely very happy to be either finished with school, starting a new job, or both. He or she perceives the employment setting and his or her new coworkers in a positive light—through "rose-colored glasses." During this phase of employment, your preceptee is actively focused on developing skills, mastering work routines, and making new friends.

The shock phase

Your preceptee will move into the shock phase if any of the following occur:

- Your preceptee encounters health care coworkers with weaknesses, such as tardiness or inattention to duty
- Your preceptee finds a lack of supplies, poor equipment maintenance, failures in communication, or other obstacles to providing excellent nursing care
- Your preceptee discovers potential inconsistencies in professional nursing behaviors

Any other situation that causes frustration, anger, embarrassment, or disillusionment could potentially send a preceptee into the shock phase. A situation that typically initiates this phase is when a preceptee is humiliated by a senior health care worker.

The recovery phase

Your preceptee can achieve the recovery phase once he or she is able to perceive the realities of the health care employment setting with a balanced view of both the positive and negative aspects. Your preceptee must establish consistent expectations for all of his or her coworkers. This is a perspective that must be learned from within the work setting. The preceptee has to realize that not all health care workers have uniform conformity to the institution's standards for conduct. Once this perspective is achieved, the preceptee may even be able to see him- or herself as fallible. During the recovery phase, a lost sense of humor may return to the preceptee.

The resolution phase

Danger lurks within the resolution phase—danger that the preceptee may adopt less-than-ideal values or beliefs in order to resolve the conflict of values with the team, and thus "fit in." Ideally, the preceptee will retain the positive aspects of his or her nursing value/belief system (i.e., the one taught at school) and the unit's (i.e., the one held by practicing nurses). This would be a realistic way to resolve the conflict.

How do you, as the preceptor, work within each of these phases to ensure that reality shock does not lead to resignation or adoption of poor values?

During the honeymoon phase, the preceptor should not misconstrue the real feelings that may be developing in the preceptee. Now is not the time for complacency, despite seemingly positive statements made by your preceptee. The initial bonds between you and your preceptee need to be developed here. These bonds are created by a mutual sense of trust, respect, and honor.

Gaining the **trust** of your preceptee involves the following:

- Ensuring that feedback is always given in private
- Not permitting gossip about your preceptee to be perpetuated
- Following through with what you have promised to do

Earning the **respect** of your preceptee involves the following:

- Not requesting your preceptee to do any task that you would not do
- Living up to the ideals of a professional nurse (uniform, appearance, breaks, interactions with others, and so on)
- Giving simple, easy-to-follow directions for tasks
- Listening carefully to all that your preceptee says
- Treating your preceptee nicely

Honor among professionals is developed by the following:

- Standing up for each other in times of adversity
- Always speaking kindly about other nursing staff
- Living the trust and respect rules

What is most important to develop between you and your preceptee, however, is clear, open communication. Although your preceptee may state that everything is "great," the preceptor needs to spend time each day with your preceptee, away from the crowd, discussing the day's events, asking how your preceptee felt, and expressing encouragement.

Despite best intentions, there are many influences on your preceptee that are beyond your control. Other staff may exhibit less-professional behaviors, less-professional dress, or a less-professional work ethic. If your preceptee observes that others can do less and experience no negative consequences, he or she may develop some disillusionment. Therefore, it is important for you to investigate whether your preceptee is experiencing these feelings. Ask some probing questions such as, "Have you noticed any behaviors among the staff that disturb you?" or "Are there any practices you have observed here on the nursing unit that you do not agree with?"

Equipment and supply issues that plague the nursing unit may affect your preceptee's perception of a professional practice environment. It is important for your preceptee to see that you take a proactive stance to solve problems. Some problem resolution during the preceptorship program may ultimately prevent your preceptee from seeing the work environment as unchangeable.

It is very important that you recognize when your preceptee is in the shock phase and continue to keep up the open communication pattern already developed.

In order to help your preceptee move toward the recovery phase, a balanced view of the workplace must be presented.

Here again, open, honest communication regarding the nursing unit must be held. The expression of your true feelings and real anecdotes about situations faced, actions contemplated, and outcomes show your preceptee that he or she too can overcome obstacles to professional practice.

Be very conscious of the potential for your preceptee to slip back into poor habits, mimicking those habits of other nurses. Your role as preceptor—to guide, to reflect, to provide feedback—must be actively engaged to prevent this.

Communication is the key to preventing reality shock from becoming a negative consequence for a new preceptee. Establishing open, honest, trusting communication from the beginning will prove to be a valuable tool.

Validating competency

Competency is the goal of the precepting process.

The preceptorship program is effective if your orientee attains competency on the required elements of the unit orientation. Competency consists of three elements: technical competence, interpersonal competence, and decision-making competence.

Competency-based orientation

A competency-based orientation focuses on the end results—

that is, the ability of a newly hired employee to perform expected job responsibilities. The emphasis is on the performance of specific responsibilities as well as the acquisition of knowledge.

This method of orientation provides structure for new employees and preceptors, because tasks and learning activities are clearly identified.

The skill and knowledge level of new employees should be evaluated before he or she begins clinical practice. This can be accomplished though shared knowledge and testing. Competency statements concentrate on what the person can do, as well as the knowledge the person has acquired. This can be accomplished through evaluation of the skills checklist, discussion, observation, or a combination of these strategies.

The three important elements of competency-based orientation are as follows:

1. Technical competence

Technical competence is the most familiar element. Elements of technical competence are traditionally found on orientation checklists.

These are the psychomotor tasks that the new employee must perform safely and effectively in order to do the job. Measure technical competence by observing how the new nurse

- draws blood from arterial line
- validates accuracy of data transfer
- identifies panic values and takes appropriate action
- responds to stat order within 30 minutes

To reach the advanced level of technical competency, add an efficiency component. In health care today, performing technical skills safely and effectively is the minimum standard. Performing these skills in a time-efficient manner with minimal supplies is also necessary.

2. **Interpersonal competence**

Interpersonal competence refers to the effective use of interpersonal communication skills when working with customers and fellow employees. Team building, conflict resolution, and customer relations are the key components of interpersonal competence. These skills can also be listed on an orientation checklist. Measure interpersonal competencies by monitoring whether your orientee

- greets patients/families with warmth
- displays proper phone etiquette
- introduces him/herself to patient and explains role
- works cooperatively with team members

In health care, interpersonal competence is more than just being courteous. Interpersonal competency stems from a caring attitude. Patients and families look for specific behaviors that convey a caring attitude. The following behaviors can also be used to monitor interpersonal competency:

- Calling the patient by his or her preferred name
- Introducing him/herself to the patient and explaining his or her role in the patient's care
- Sitting down, at eye level, and collaboratively planning or reviewing care
- Touching the patient or family member in the form of a handshake, handholding, a comforting pat on the shoulder, and so on
- Anticipating patient and family needs for information, pain relief, bathroom, or food and fluids by having needed items readily accessible
- Expecting patient and family anxiety and offering information, reassurance and comfort as appropriate

3. Decision-making competence

Decision-making competence is manifested in the new employee's ability to apply the principles of critical thinking and problem solving to decision making. Your orientee assess facts, recognize problems, identify alternative actions, anticipate outcomes, and make choices. Effective decision-making is predicated on the ability to think critically.

Critical thinking involves asking questions to get beneath the surface of a problem. Unlike traditional thinking, which tends to preserve the status quo, critical thinking generates more questions and, as a result, increases the number of possible solutions.

Critical thinking is a skill that can be learned. The mind is a pattern-making system. It creates, stores, and recognizes patterns. We learn by assimilating experiences and grouping them into ordered patterns.

Many times, you'll need to generate a lot of ideas to come up with a few that will solve the problem. The problems in health care are usually complex, and they seldom have one right solution. Challenge your orientee to think beyond the obvious right answer and identify additional "right" answers.

Questions to promote critical thinking

- Given these lab results, how will you change your nursing care plan?
- How will you prioritize your plan today?
- What other alternative nursing measures would work?
- How will you determine the effectiveness of that intervention?

Distinguishing competencies

Keep in mind the following:

- Competency is more than just a skill, such as setting up a patient-controlled analgesia (PCA) pump. Competency is setting up a PCA pump, programming it according to a physician's orders, and monitoring the effect on the patient.

- Competency is not just having knowledge, such as being able to identify ventricular tachycardia on an ECG rhythm strip. Competency is identifying ventricular tachycardia on an ECG rhythm strip, assessing the hemodynamic effect of the rhythm on the patient, intervening appropriately and in accordance with unit policy or a physician's orders, and reassessing the patient to ensure that planned interventions are appropriate.

- Competency is not just good behavior, such as addressing the patient by his or her preferred name. Competency is consistently demonstrating a caring attitude, which includes addressing the patient by his or her preferred name, answering the patient's call bell in a timely manner, and not leaving the patient's room without finding out whether there is anything else the patient needs.

Competency can be measured against well-developed professional standards published by organizations such as the state board of nursing, a professional nursing organization, or the Joint Commission on Accreditation of Healthcare Organizations.

Competency also can be improved through training and development. In any clinical environment, staff may have the knowledge, the skills, and the good behaviors, but can they use these to do the job? That is validation of their competency. Therefore, one of your major roles is to validate the competency of your preceptee prior to the end of the preceptorship program.

You must avoid the trap of confusing competency with the traits and characteristics of your preceptee. Personality descriptors and distinguishing qualities are not performance indicators. The following is a list of some common traits that you should *not* use to evaluate competency:

cooperative	conforms to policies
assertive	independent
committed	shows initiative
decisive	flexible
creative	is a team player

Personality traits such as those listed above are formed early in life. During the preceptorship program, do not focus energy on trying to change or develop them. Nor should you base the evaluation of clinical competency on these traits.

Providing feedback

Providing ongoing evaluation of your orientee is essential. Your orientee needs daily feedback on the things he or she is doing well, areas in which additional work is needed, and progress toward orientation goals.

Daily feedback allows you to do the following:

- Motivate and positively reinforce learning
- Diagnose the nature and extent of any problems

- Offer constructive criticism
- Identify areas in need of remediation
- Determine the effectiveness of the learning experience

We have all received comments such as "good job," or "nice work." Such comments make us feel good, but they do not tell us what we have achieved, accomplished, or produced that was "good" or "nice." When giving feedback, be objective and specific.

Facilitate learning and prevent the destruction of ego by developing effective feedback techniques.

BEER feedback method

One technique for creating effective feedback is to use the following four-step model for criticizing and correcting behavior and performance problems.

This model is based on a process that involves asking yourself questions about your precptee's behavior. Remember the acronym "BEER":

B: Behavior—What is it the employee is doing or not doing that is unacceptable?

E: Effect—Why is the behavior unacceptable? How does it hurt productivity, bother others, and so on?

E: Expectation—What is it you expect the employee to do or not to do to change?

R: Result—What will happen if the employee changes (positive tone) or this behavior continues (negative tone)?

Once you've formulated your feedback, use the following rules as guidance on giving that effective feedback to your preceptee:

Use descriptive terms rather than evaluative terms.
Always make a conscious effort to describe both positive and negative behaviors.

For example, you observe your preceptee greeting the patient correctly and stating that she was her nurse for the day and what her name was. However, your preceptee did not have on her nametag. Rather than saying to her, "Your name tag is missing, and the manager won't like that!" (an evaluation), it would be better to say, "You greeted that patient according to the unit guidelines. Can you think of anything that would help your patient remember you?"

Be specific rather than general in comments. Anecdotal records that you use to discuss progress should be very specific regarding observed behaviors or skills.

For example, your preceptee had learned to successfully initiate intravenous (IV) therapy this past week. A general comment in your preceptee's weekly anecdotal record might be, "IV initiation skills acceptable." A more specific comment would be, "Preceptee initiated three IV starts with a single attempt each time, aseptic technique used, and patients stated that process was comfortable."

Focus on your preceptee's behavior rather than on his or her personality. Anecdotal records should not reflect personality conflicts between you and your preceptee or your preceptee and other staff. However, behaviors that need to be corrected need to have focused comments related to those behaviors, not the personality traits displayed behind the behavior.

For example, your preceptee has been consistently late for the patient report at the beginning of the shift. She disrupts the shift report when she comes in late, and the rest of the staff has complained to you of this rude, disruptive behavior. They say she is inconsiderate.

A comment with a personality-based focus is, "You have been very inconsiderate of the other staff members. They don't like you interrupting report."

A comment with a behavior-based focus is, "You have been arriving at report late this week. Is there a problem arriving on time? When a staff member is late, it disrupts the flow of the report and items may be missed. What can you do to ensure that you are here on time? "

Focus on sharing information rather than giving advice. For example, saying, "I think that you (the preceptee) should do Mrs. Jones' dressing now, as she is scheduled for physio at 1500" is giving advice. But saying, "I just got a call from physio; Mrs. Jones is scheduled for 1500. Is there anything she needs done prior to her appointment?" is sharing information.

Feedback should be well-timed. A case of poorly timed feedback: You observe a mistake in transcription of a physician order while at the nursing station, and you tell your preceptee in front of the unit clerk that the error has been made and to correct it.

To provide well-timed feedback, remove the chart to the break room where no one is present, and there you tell your preceptee that the error has been made and to correct it.

Give your preceptee enough time to accept the feedback prior to making a plan that will involve a change in behavior. For example, an impatient preceptor would say, "You consistently fail to listen to all areas of the anterior and posterior chest when doing your respiratory assessment. What are you going to do about it?" But a patient preceptor would give the preceptee time by saying, "You consistently fail to listen to all areas of the anterior and posterior chest when doing your respiratory assessment. Please review the assessment process in your text and get back to me tomorrow about how you can use this information to improve."

Avoid giving the impression that you and other staff are "ganging up" on your preceptee. An example of ganging-up is saying, "The staff and I feel that you are spending too much time with the patients and not enough time completing your charting." One way to say this without giving the impression of ganging up is to say, "I have observed you spending a lot of time with the patients, but noticed your documentation has not been complete."

Evaluations

Evaluations should be affirming and future-oriented. It is important to identify things that are positive and encouraging. Also identify what has been accomplished and suggest ways to build on those areas in the future. Evaluations should be educational and enhance self-esteem.

There should not be any surprises in evaluations if you have been giving daily feedback and opportunity to correct behaviors.

As each required competency is successfully demonstrated, tell your orientee that an objective has been completed. Review the documentation form each day and check off the day's accomplishments. This exercise helps your orientee identify progress and feel successful.

It is also important to communicate to your orientee the areas that need further experience or improvement. Be direct and address negatives first. Do not sandwich negatives between two positives; that approach dilutes the effectiveness of both. Do not be apologetic about constructive criticism. As a preceptor, you have both a right and a responsibility to require good performance.

Collaborate with your orientee to develop a plan to improve these areas. Areas for improvement must be discussed as they are identified. Don't wait until the last day of orientation to tell your orientee everything he or she is not doing correctly. Also, keep the manager updated on any areas that are failing to progress as expected.

Do the following when you sit down with your orientee for an evaluation:

- Find a quiet, controlled environment without interruptions
- Maintain a relaxed but professional atmosphere
- Put your orientee at ease
- Review specific examples of both positive and negative behaviors
- Discuss future needs and goals
- Express confidence in his or her ability to do the work
- Be sincere and constructive in both praise and criticism
- Ask your orientee how you, as preceptor, can improve the learning experience

End of orientation evaluation

At the end of orientation, you will prepare a written evaluation of your orientee's performance. Review this written documentation with the manager before sharing it with your orientee. The final evaluation is a summary of the daily evaluations you have had with your orientee. There should be no information in the final evaluation that you haven't already discussed with your orientee in a more informal setting.

During this final evaluation, allow time for your orientee to provide verbal and written comments on your evaluation. Also ask him or her to evaluate the orientation process and your effectiveness as a preceptor. Ask for his or her input on how to make things better for the next orientee.

It is your responsibility to bring closure to the preceptee-orientee relationship and initiate the peer relationship. The new status of your orientee should be clearly communicated to him or her and to the team. A simple and effective way of signaling the change in relationship is to say to your orientee, "I've enjoyed being your preceptor, and I'm looking forward to working with you." For the staff, an equally simple and direct approach is to announce, "This is Sandy's last day of orientation," or "This is Sandy's first day off orientation."

You may want to initiate a simple ceremony or recognition for the new employee. This can take the form of a certificate of completion, presented on the first day after orientation in front of the staff. Another strategy is to plan a group lunch/dinner in honor of the new staff member. Any strategy that conveys your orientee's change of status and welcomes him or her to the team is appropriate.

Final exam

1. A learning style inventory test reveals that your orientee is a tactile learner. Which of the following would likely be the most effective way to teach him or her about the unit's admission database?

   a. Give the orientee a printout of instructions that he or she can use to follow along.
   b. Let the orientee enter sample patient data into the database as you explain it.
   c. Use a PowerPoint slide presentation to walk your orientee through the process.
   d. all of the above

2. Which skill-based domain of learning is best described by the terms imitation, practice, and habit?

   a. psychomotor domain
   b. cognitive domain
   c. affective domain
   d. none of the above

3. The author describes a unit's emotional climate for learning as "a comfort zone, where everyone understands that every person's views are valued and respected as equal." What way does the author suggest you test the emotional climate for learning on your unit?

   a. Conduct an anonymous poll of unit staff.
   b. Let your preceptee introduce him- or herself to the other unit team members.

c. Ask your manager to conduct a staff evaluation.

d. Encourage your preceptee to bring up a subject or an idea for discussion during a staff meeting.

4. **Giving daily feedback to your preceptee allows you to do which of the following:**

   a. Motivate and positively reinforce learning.

   b. Diagnose the nature and extent of any problems.

   c. Determine the effectiveness of the learning experience.

   d. all of the above

5. **The best way to prevent a new nurse from resigning due to "reality shock," is by establishing clear, open communication with him or her during the first of the four phases of workplace acclimation. The name of that first phase is:**

   a. the shock phase

   b. the recovery phase

   c. the honeymoon phase

   d. the resolution phase

6. **Which of the following could you observe to validate, or measure, a preceptee's technical competence?**

   a. The way your preceptee draws blood from an arterial line.

   b. Your preceptee's greeting technique when taking on a new patient.

   c. Your preceptee's ability to be on time for report.

   d. The number of times your preceptee uses critical thinking to solve problems.

7. Which of the following does the author suggest is an effective way to introduce your preceptee to the rest of the unit?

  a. A welcome tea is held for the staff.
  b. A brief biography, written by the preceptee, is posted on the nursing unit welcome board.
  c. A picture of the preceptee is posted on the nursing unit's bulletin board.
  d. all of the above

8. During the end of the orientation evaluation, you mention to your orientee that since the first day of orientation her discharge documentation has been incomplete. What fundamental rule of the final evaluation have you forgotten?

9. Competency consists of what three elements?

10. What is the significance of the saying, "Thou shalt not make a clone of thyself"?

Answers to the final exam

1. B   2. A
3. D   4. D
5. C   6. A
7. D

8. There should be no surprises during the final evaluation. Instead, it should be a summary of the daily feedback you've been giving to your orientee.

9. Technical competence, interpersonal competence, and decision-making competence

10. This is a quick reminder that the way you may have learned how to do something isn't the only way a process can be done. If a student learns another way of doing a task, yet the end result is the same, you should be satisfied. Remember that there's more than one way to get something done.

CERTIFICATE OF COMPLETION

This is to certify that

_____

has read and successfully passed the final exam of

The Effective Nurse Preceptor Handbook: Your guide to success

Suzanne Perney

Suzanne Perney
Vice President/Publisher